D0329041

Jane Harris
55 W Montrose Av
South Orange NJ 0'

WITHDRAWN

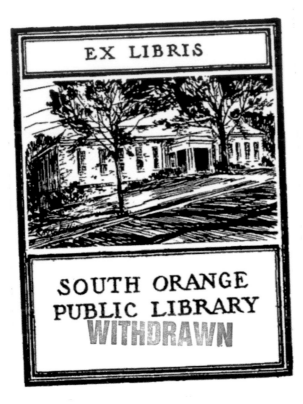

Yoga in an Adirondack Chair

Yoga in an Adirondack Chair

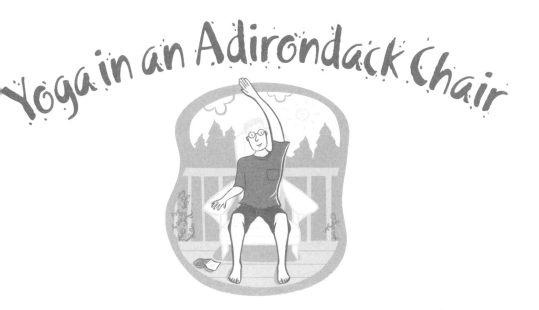

A GUIDE FOR EVERYONE

CAROL SHERMAN AND SUSAN FEATHERS

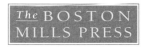

The BOSTON MILLS PRESS

A SMITH SHERMAN BOOK

National Library of Canada Cataloguing in Publication Data
Sherman, Carol, 1950–

Yoga in an Adirondack chair
Issued also under title: Yoga in a Muskoka chair.

ISBN 1-55046-341-1

1. Yoga, Hatha   I. Feathers, Susan, 1961–   II. Title.

RA781.7.F416 2001a   613.7'046   C2001–930104–9

05 04 03 02 01   1 2 3 4 5

Published in 2001 by Boston Mills Press
132 Main Street, Erin, Ontario, N0B 1T0
Tel 519-833-2407   Fax 519-833-2195
e-mail books@bostonmillspress.com
www.bostonmillspress.com

An affiliate of Stoddart Publishing Co. Limited
895 Don Mills Road
400-2 Park Centre
Toronto, Ontario, Canada, M3c 1W3
Tel 416-445-3333   Fax 416-445-5967
e-mail gdsinc@genpub.com

Distributed in Canada by
General Distribution Services Limited
325 Humber College Boulevard
Toronto, Ontario, M9W 7C3
Orders 1-800-387-0141 Ontario & Quebec
Orders 1-800-387-0172 NW Ontario
& other provinces
e-mail cservice@genpub.com

Distributed in the United States by
General Distribution Services Inc.
PMB 128, 4500 Witmer Industrial Estates
Niagara Falls, New York 14305-1386
Toll-free 1-800-805-1083
Toll-free fax 1-800-481-6207
e-mail gdsinc@genpub.com
www.genpub.com

Design and page composition by PageWave Graphics Inc.

Printed in Canada by Friesen Printers

*We acknowledge for their financial support of our publishing program the Canada Council,
the Ontario Arts Council, and the Government of Canada through the Book Publishing Industry
Development Program (BPIDP).*

To Erik and Jakob
C.S.

To the memory of my first guru: my father
S.F.

Contents

Introduction

If you think yoga is weird positions and threading string up your nose, you're only partly right. It's true that many of yoga's more advanced postures may seem slightly strange, what with legs wrapped around the body and arms every which way — and there is an exercise to clear the nose that does involve string. (We're not going to teach you that one, though.) Generally, yoga is a system of physical and mental exercises designed to balance and unite the body and mind. Anyone can do it. We thought it would be great to combine yoga with the unique design of an Adirondack chair. So with just a little bit of a stretch, nirvana will be yours.

Yoga started somewhere in India about 6,000 years ago. The most popular type of yoga in the West — and the focus of this book — is Hatha yoga, which combines breathing, postures and concentration exercises. Although the Adirondack chair hasn't been around anywhere near as long (less than 100 years), its design principles are perfectly suited to yoga. With its slightly sloping back and its wide Popeye-like arms, the Adirondack chair provides an ideal starting point. The stillness and stability that are the essence of an effective yoga practice can be experienced perfectly in the grounded and comfortable Adirondack chair. Of course, the postures can be easily modified for any chair, but we recommend that you first try the Adirondack chair if you can.

In this little book, you'll find a breath for when you're feeling unhinged and lots of warm-up exercises, including one of our favorites, an ear arousal that's guaranteed to get you going. Traditional yoga postures such as the Fish and Cobra are here, except you get to do them in a chair. There's a candle-gazing meditation, and if you're inclined to get up there's an Out of Chair Experience chapter with exercises that can be done standing or lying on the cottage dock. There's even a section of Menus, specially designed routines including Energizer, Relaxer and Quickie. Self-explanatory, no?

If you're interested in maintaining good physical health and calming a busy mind, follow the simple routine in this guide. You'll see definite improvement after only a short time of practice. All of the exercises have been reviewed for accuracy and safety by a certified yoga teacher with 15 years of experience. Whatever your goal — toning your body, relieving stress or gaining peace of mind — yoga will help you attain it. So take a deep breath, sit back and begin. The benefits are amazing.

Easy Pose

This is perhaps the only place you'll ever get instructions on how to sit in an Adirondack chair. Yoga takes no pose for granted. This pose is really easy. That's why we've called it Easy Pose. This is your basic sitting posture. Assume it at the beginning and end of each exercise. It's great for the breathing exercises, many of the postures and perfect for meditation.

- Place your feet flat on the ground, about shoulder width apart.
- Place drink, book, magazine or Game Boy™ on the ground.
- Relax your arms along the arms of the chair with your palms facing down.
- Rest back and shoulder blades against the back of the chair.
- Head should not rest against chair.
- Relax shoulders.
- Look forward.

BE MINDFUL

If you are a beginner, you will probably want to keep your eyes open, but as yoga becomes more familiar, you may want to close them. It's a good start to meditation.

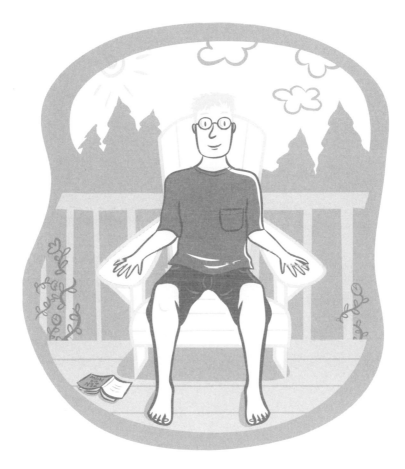

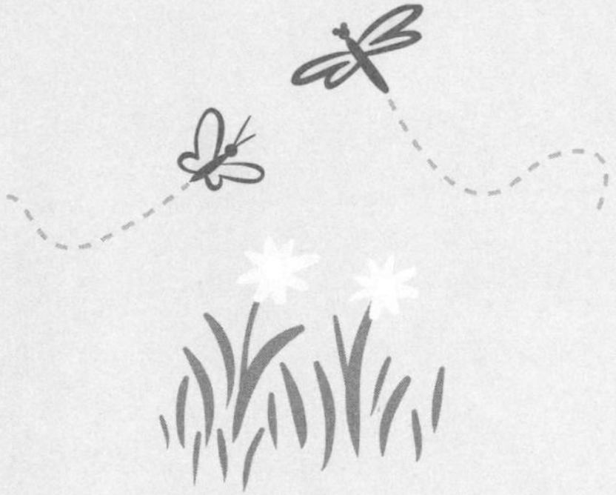

Breathing

Breathing

The most important ingredient in any exercise is the breath. Most people skimp on the air they breathe and don't even know it. Shallow breathing causes the body to release an array of hormones that are quite useful if you're preparing for battle or running away in terror from a bean sprout sandwich. But if that is how you normally feed your body oxygen, it will eventually cause chronic stress, insomnia or depression.

If you often feel anxious for no apparent reason, you are likely breathing improperly. It takes a little practice, but once you've got the proper method down, your mind will be sharper and your body more relaxed.

Breathing Primer

First, take a long, deep breath through your nose, expanding your stomach. Pause for a moment, then exhale through the nose and let your stomach fall inward. In time, you will notice that your upper chest and lower chest also rise and fall with your breath. When you are doing yoga postures, focus on your breath to release tension in any particularly tight area. Proper breathing is essential.

In life, when faced with a difficult situation, trauma or stress, remember to use your breath to bring calmness to your mind and body. We can face almost any obstacle with equanimity and inspired thoughtfulness when we breathe fully and deeply.

BE MINDFUL

Don't strain the muscles of your face.

Relax your jaw.

Relax your neck and shoulders.

Stop if you feel lightheaded.

Alternating Breath

When you're feeling stressed or unhinged, Alternating Breath is a perfect way to bring you back to your wonderful balanced self. If your nasal passages are too congested, then sit this one out. Also, tradition dictates you use your right hand throughout the exercise.

- Sit comfortably in Easy Pose.
- Close your right nostril with your right thumb.
- Inhale through your left nostril to a count of four.
- Gently press your ring finger against the left nostril, so that both nostrils are closed. Hold the breath to a count of 12.
- Continue to close your left nostril while releasing your right. Exhale to a count of eight.
- Inhale through your right nostril to a count of four.
- Gently press your thumb against the right nostril, so that both nostrils are closed. Hold the breath to a count of 12.
- Continue to close the right nostril while releasing your ring finger from the left. Exhale to a count of eight.
- Repeat the cycle up to eight times.

BE MINDFUL
Keep your elbow down and shoulders relaxed.

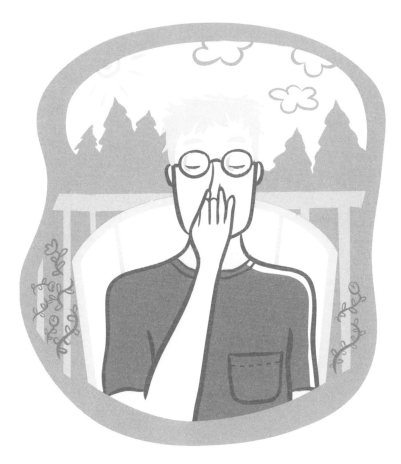

Breath of Fire

You could also call this Hard-to-Explain Breath. Breath of Fire is a great way to start the day. It's a series of rapid, forceful abdominal breaths that have an energizing effect. As an added bonus, it also tones your abdomen.

- Sit comfortably in Easy Pose or lean slightly forward.

- Inhale slowly and deeply through both nostrils.

- Pull your abdominal muscles inward sharply and forcefully exhale through the nostrils.

- Immediately release your abdomen and let a natural inhalation occur. Don't hold your breath. Then forcefully exhale again.

- Do 10 to 15 of these quick pumping breaths. More with practice.

- Make the last exhalation in the series a slow one.

- After one round take two deep breaths. Take a third comfortable breath and retain for 20 seconds. Gradually build up to a one-minute retention. You may experience a lightheadedness.

- Practice three rounds of Breath of Fire.

BE MINDFUL

Belly should expand as you breathe in and contract as you breathe out.

WARNING: Do not retain breath if you have high blood pressure.

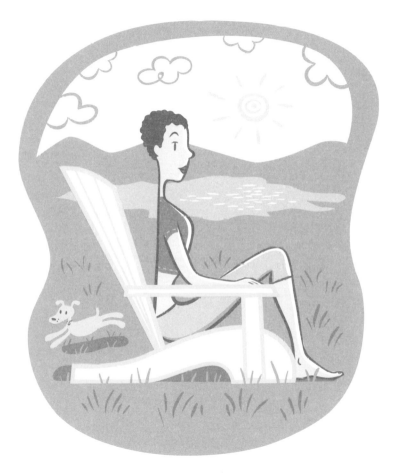

Cooling Breath

This exercise is great if you're stranded on a desert island or relaxing during a heat wave at the cottage and you've run out of beer, oops, soy milk. Not only does Cooling Breath reduce thirst, it releases tension in the neck and head and has a cooling effect on the body. So turn your tongue into a straw and suck air. It's one of the only times in yoga that you inhale through your mouth rather than your nose.

- Sit comfortably in Easy Pose.
- Close your eyes and stick your tongue straight out, curling the outer edges upward as much as you can. (It's easier to curl your tongue if it's not out too far.)
- Suck air in through your tongue.
- Exhale slowly through your nose as you bring your tongue into your mouth.
- Repeat up to two more times.

BE MINDFUL

Don't do this exercise if you're chilly or start to feel cold while doing. Do only two to three cycles.

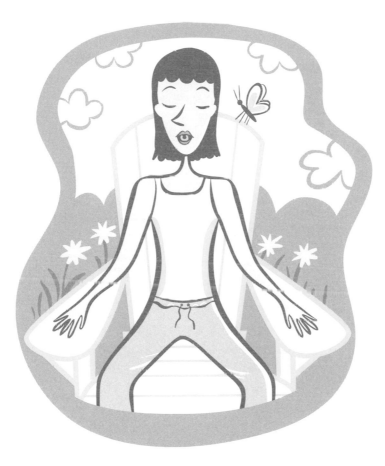

Lion Breath

One of the really neat things about yoga is how many of the postures are named after animals. In this facial exercise you get to roar like a lion and stick out your tongue. Be aggressive and really roar. Oh yeah, one other thing. You might want to warn people what you're up to. The Lion helps you relieve tension in the facial muscles, especially the jaw, and is particularly helpful with a cough or sore throat.

- Sit comfortably in Easy Pose. (After you inhale deeply through your nose, do the rest of the moves simultaneously.)
- Inhale deeply.
- Open your mouth wide and as you exhale stick your tongue out, trying to touch your chin, and roar from the back of your throat.
- Open your eyes wide — a subtle movement, just thinking wide will do it. Don't wrinkle your brow. Hindus roll their eyes back into their heads, but maybe that's a little too Boris Karloff for you.
- If you really want to get into it, place your palms on your knees, and gently lean into your hands and spread your fingers wide.

BE MINDFUL

Be gentle. Don't overextend. Especially watch the neck, leave it in neutral.

Don't repeat more than three breaths.

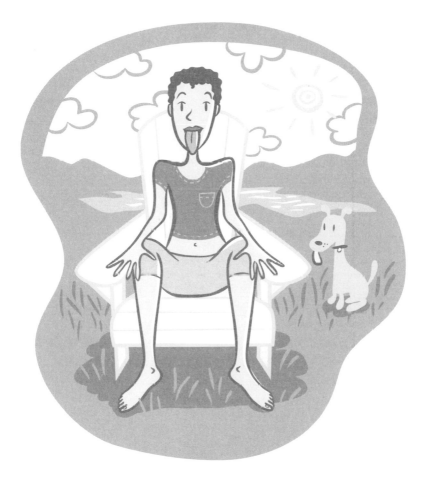

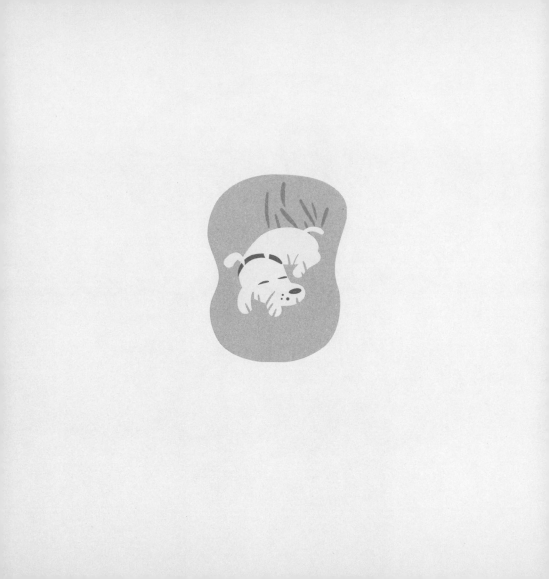

Warm-Ups

Warm-Ups

Someone we know likes to have a bath to warm-up for her
warm-ups. A hot summer day is good, too. While warm baths and
sweat are good, it is still important to limber up inactive muscles
with gentle warm-ups before beginning any of the postures. Many
people skip warm-ups completely because they don't have the
time or think they aren't necessary. Think again, Kemo Swami.
You will obtain the maximum benefit from yoga, or any exercise
you do, if you warm up first. When your muscles and joints are
warmed-up, the benefits will increase. Your range of motion
expands and you perform the postures more effectively, avoiding
soreness and injury.

After completing a few breathing exercises, these simple
sitting stretches will prepare you for the poses. Each stretch helps
to relieve tension in a particular body part. The Mountain, for
instance, focuses on the arms and shoulders; Neck Rolls release
tension in the shoulder and neck muscles; the Eye Exercises relax
the facial muscles.

Be sure to breathe slowly and rhythmically throughout all of the warm-ups. Focus on the muscles being stretched and never extend beyond what is comfortable. Remember to take your time with each exercise and hold each warm-up only as long as it feels good.

BE MINDFUL

Don't bounce. Pulsing movements only add to your risk of muscle tears and soreness.

Don't stretch to the point of pain. "No pain, no gain" is a myth. Throw it into the lake with your cellphone.

Don't hold your breath.

Mountain

You don't have to leave your chair or put on hiking boots to climb this mountain. Yogis think of this pose as one that teaches stability and grounding. This simple warm-up will limber up and tone your arms and shoulders, deepen your breathing and strengthen your spine.

- Sit comfortably in Easy Pose.
- Place the palms of your hands together in front of your chest in a "prayer" position.
- Take one deep inhalation and exhalation.
- Inhale again and, keeping your palms together, slowly move the arms above your head. Let your hands separate slightly with palms facing each other.
- Stretch your fingers up to the sky. Feel your spine lengthen.
- Hold this position for up to 10 seconds.
- Exhale and come down exactly the way you went up, returning your hands to the original "prayer" position in front of your chest.
- Repeat three times.

BE MINDFUL

Don't hunch your shoulders.

Feel the stretch in your shoulder blades.

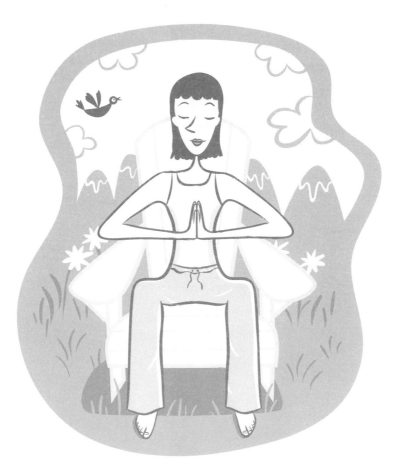

Flower

What could be more magical and beautiful than the slow unfurling of a flower's petals? In this exercise, nature is in your hands. This position will stretch, tone and strengthen your hands, wrists and arms, and improve circulation. For late bloomers everywhere.

- Sit comfortably in Easy Pose.
- Lift your arms straight out in front of you to shoulder height. Keep elbows straight and hands in front of you, palms down and shoulders relaxed.
- Make tight fists with your hands.
- Slowly unfold your hands imagining they are flowers.
- Stretch the fingers as far apart as possible.
- Make a tight fist again.
- Release and return to Easy Pose.
- Repeat three times.

BE MINDFUL

Don't raise your arms too high.

Don't be too rigid.

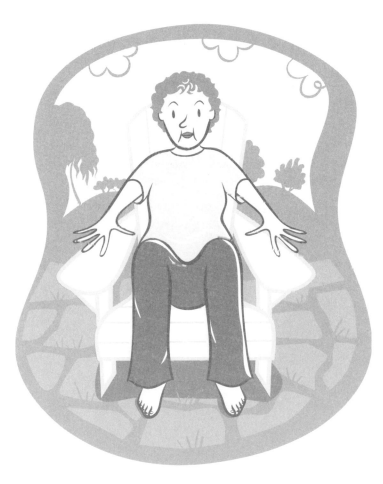

Neck Rolls

This warm-up exercise is a classic, whether you're practicing yoga, aerobics or bench pressing. These simple neck exercises relax the head and limber up the neck and shoulder muscles.

- Sit comfortably in Easy Pose.
- Allow your head to sink gently forward toward your chest without forcing or straining.
- Inhale and slowly and gently guide your chin to the right over the chest until the head is completely lifted and you are gazing over the right shoulder.
- Exhale and slowly and gently take the same path back to center.
- Inhale and repeat on the other side.
- Repeat as often as you like — the slower the better.

BE MINDFUL

Don't overdo the stretch. Be gentle, never strain.

Be sure to move very slowly throughout this exercise.

Keep your shoulders relaxed.

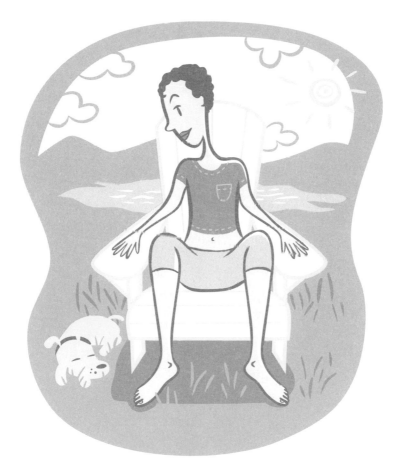

Eye Exercises

You'll look a little shifty-eyed doing this first exercise, but it not only strengthens your eye muscles, it gives you a bright-eyed feeling, too. Remember to keep your head still and your facial muscles relaxed as you do the eye movements. The Eye Warmer relaxes and soothes the eyes after the circle exercise.

EYE CIRCLES

- Looking straight ahead, imagine a large clock (much bigger than your face) with the numbers right in front of your eyes.

- Look at 12 o'clock.

- Without moving your head, let your eyes glide slowly in one continuous motion from 12 to 1 o'clock, 2 o'clock, etc., until you return to 12. (This exercise will take about 30 seconds.)

- Repeat the exercise in a counterclockwise direction starting at 12 and gliding to 11 o'clock, 10 o'clock, etc.

EYE WARMER

- Vigorously rub the palms of your hands together. (They should feel warm and tingly.)

- Place the heels of your palms gently over your closed eyelids.

- Hold for 10 seconds.

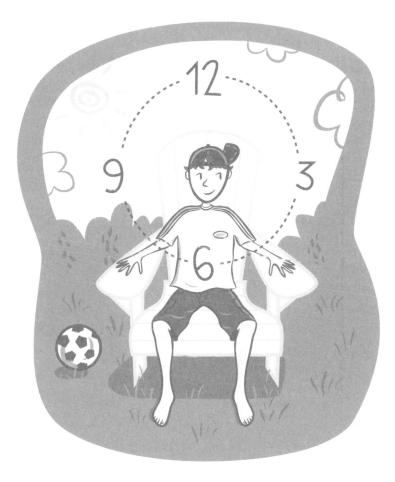

Ear Massage

Anyone who has ever gotten a reaction by kissing someone's ear could tell you what a stimulating place the earlobe is. No, we're not asking you to kiss your own ears here. This is a finger-to-ear rub to arouse the nerve endings. Hold the romance for the double leg lifts!

- Hold the bottom of your earlobes with your thumbs and index fingers.
- Move slowly up and down your outer ears, lightly pinching.
- Return to the bottom of your earlobes and apply gentle pressure to both ears for 15 seconds.

BE MINDFUL
You might want to remove any earrings first.

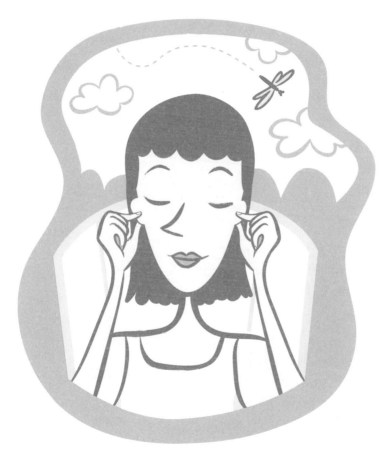

Leg Exercises

We know this is going to sound unbelievable, especially with all the exercise we do to keep our legs and stomach in shape, but with this warm-up all you have to do is sit in the chair and lift your legs, and voilà — a flat stomach and toned legs.

SINGLE LEG LIFTS

- Sit comfortably in Easy Pose.
- Inhale and slowly straighten your right knee and lift your leg until it is straight out in front of you at about hip level. Reach your toes upward and push heels away from your body.
- Hold for one breath.
- Exhale and slowly lower your leg to a count of four.
- Repeat with left leg. Do three lifts with each leg, alternating legs.

DOUBLE LEG LIFTS

- Sit comfortably in Easy Pose.
- Inhale and slowly straighten both your knees and lift both legs until they are straight out in front of you at about hip level.
- Hold for one breath.
- Exhale and slowly lower your legs to a count of four.
- Repeat five to 10 times.

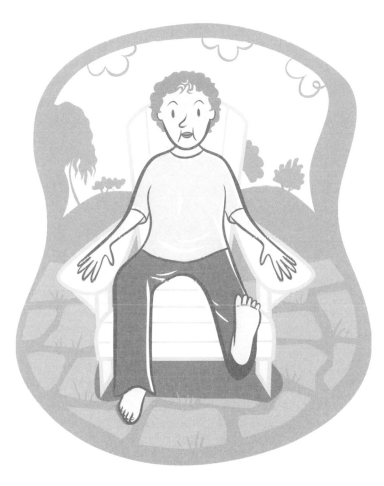

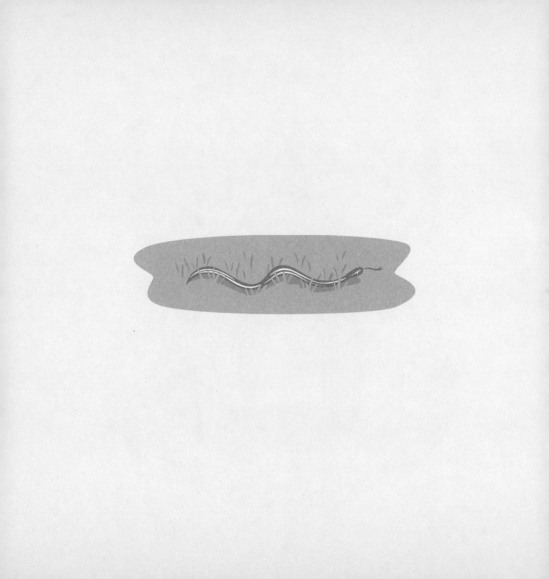

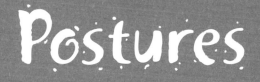

Postures

Nobody wants to get old and creaky. After only the briefest of time practicing yoga, "flexible and ageless" will be your mantra. We're not asking you to contort yourself or stand on your head (we're in a chair, for heaven's sake!). These simple but powerful poses will strengthen your body, improve spinal suppleness, tone muscles and calm your mind. Yoga hasn't survived for 6,000 years for nothing.

The postures are characterized by four basic movements: backward bending, forward bending, twisting and side stretching. There's even one where you don't do much of anything but relax. If you do the entire sequence of poses described in this chapter, you will receive a balanced workout that stretches and aligns the entire body. Although the poses are not aerobic in nature, they do send oxygen to the cells in your body through sustained stretching of your different muscle groups.

Try to follow the postures in the sequence presented here, or at least close to it. Each posture counterbalances the previous one. So if you do the Fish, for instance, where you extend backwards, be sure to follow this with the Forward Bend. Stretch gently into each position — never ever force or hold a posture if it feels uncomfortable. Listen to your body, it will help guide you.

BE MINDFUL

Begin each routine with several warm-ups.

Move slowly into each posture to avoid injury.

Don't hold your breath.

Never force or push yourself.

Smile — even the faintest one will help you relax.

Seated Relaxation

You're seated. You're relaxed. What else do you need to know!

- Sit comfortably in Easy Pose. This time, if you like, rest your head against the back of the chair and adjust your legs slightly forward.

- Close your eyes and keep them closed throughout the relaxation.

- Inhale deeply and shrug your shoulders towards your ears.

- Exhale and release your shoulders.

- Inhale and raise both arms and hands out in front of you. Make fists with your hands and release.

- Exhale and drop your arms along the arms of the chair.

- Relax your abdomen and chest by taking a deep inhalation and exhalation.

- Inhale and tip your head slightly to the right, moving your right ear to your right shoulder.

- Exhale and return to center.

- Inhale and repeat on other side.

- Scrunch your face by tightly squeezing your eyes and pursing your lips. Don't worry about what you look like. You look weird. Relax.

- Sit quietly and focus your attention on your breathing.

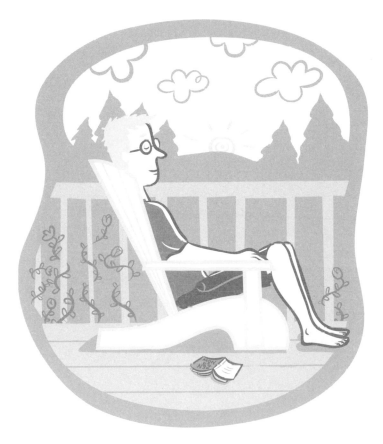

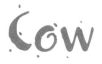

Cow

We're still working on the headstand in a chair, but we have managed to come up with a modified shoulder stand. Yoga aficionados say the shoulder stand is the "queen of postures." This seated Cow stretch essentially works many of the same muscles as the traditional posture and is an excellent overall upper body stretch. Why a cow? We have no idea. Some things in yoga remain mysterious.

- Sit comfortably in Easy Pose, but lean slightly forward.
- Inhale and rest your left arm against your back. Your elbow is bent and your palm is facing outward.
- Exhale and stretch your right arm up with the inside of your elbow beside your ear.
- Bend your elbow and reach your right hand back and try to grasp your left hand.
- Hold for one breath.
- Release and repeat on the opposite side.

BE MINDFUL

Stretch only as far as you can. Don't twist to try and clasp hands.

Relax your shoulders.

One side of your body may be more flexible than the other.

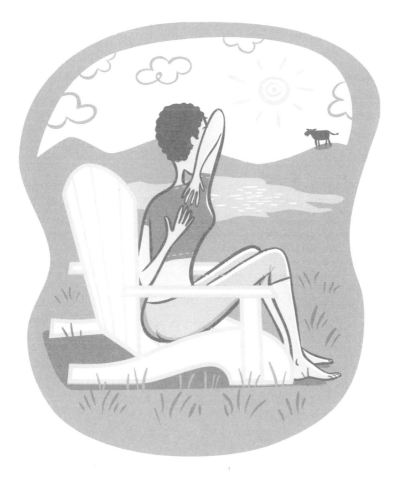

Fish

We don't want to hear any carping about this exercise. It's an intermediate posture and you may want to wriggle out of it. As in all yoga exercises, only do what is comfortably possible. This modified version of the Fish pose, a yoga classic, is a great stretch for the neck and upper and middle back. Take advantage of this position, where the chest is elevated, to take deep, energizing breaths. The chair gives a nice tilt to the legs, which will jumpstart the position.

- Sit comfortably in Easy Pose.
- Inhale and press on your elbows and forearms.
- Arch your back while pushing your chest forward.
- Drop your head back gently toward the chair and, if you can, rest the crown of your head on the back of the chair.
- Breath deeply and expand your rib cage with each inhalation.
- Hold the position for three to six breaths.
- If you really want to get into it, arch your chest even further.
- To come out of the position, very carefully lift your head and return to Easy Pose.

BE MINDFUL
Only go as far as you comfortably can. Don't overextend.

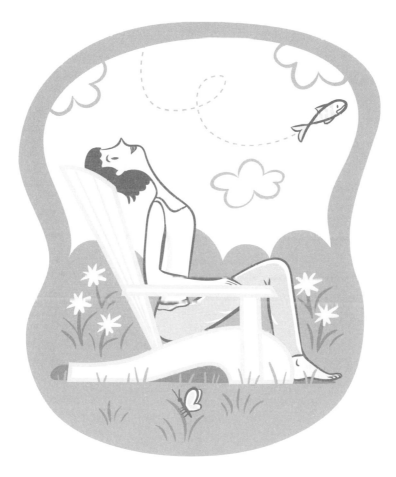

Seated Cobra

Naming a posture after the venomous frog-eating cobra seems an odd choice by the genteel vegetarian yogis of old. What were they thinking? We're sure it's because your raised head is meant to resemble the snake. Cobra in a chair strengthens the abdominal and back muscles. (For the full-length version, see page 70.) It's a great stretch, however you do it, and it helps increase circulation and improve digestion.

- Sit comfortably in Easy Pose.
- Inhale and, bending from the hips, stretch the body forward.
- Exhale and bring your chest to your knees if you can.
- Gently press your forearms along the arms of the chair and push the chest forward and lift your head.
- Hold the pose for three to six breaths.
- Exhale and release.

BE MINDFUL

Keep your shoulders down.

Shoulder blades should be flat against the back.

Don't apply too much weight to your arms. You should be able to lift your hands from the chair and maintain the pose.

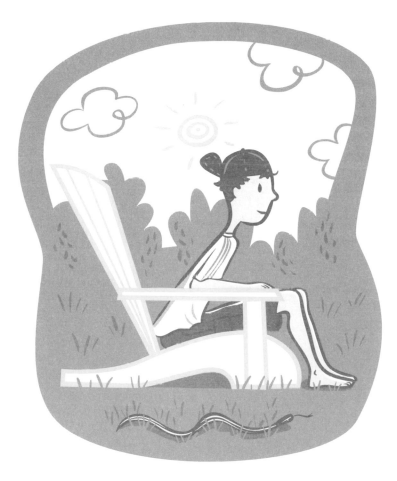

Forward Bend

Remember complaining in gym class when you had to bend over and touch your toes? You probably didn't realize then what a powerful stretch you were getting or that the Forward Bend was and is a classic yoga posture. It's a great way to release tension in your lower back.

- Sit comfortably in Easy Pose.
- Inhale and stretch your arms overhead with palms facing forward.
- Exhale and bend forward from the hips, stretching your chest over your thighs. You may be able to rest your chest right on your thighs.
- Reach forward with your arms and fingers outstretched. Keep your head parallel with your arms.
- Stay in this position for a few breaths. Then exhale and drop your head and arms gently into a ragdoll-like pose. Rest in this position for a few breaths.
- Inhale and slowly roll up vertebra by vertebra (or place your hands on your knees and slowly push yourself up).

BE MINDFUL

Only go as far as comfortably possible. Don't force your chest down. Bend at the hips, not at the middle of your back.

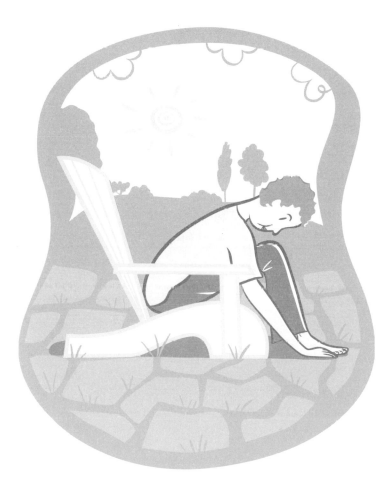

Spinal Twist

This is the perfect posture to follow the Forward Bend. The Spinal Twist provides an excellent lateral stretch for the arms, back, shoulder and neck muscles. It realigns the spine and adds flexibility to the back.

- Sit comfortably in Easy Pose.
- Place your right hand on the outside of your left knee.
- Lean slightly forward and place your left hand behind your back in any comfortable position that pulls the left arm back a little.
- On an exhale, turn your head and upper torso toward the left and look over your left shoulder.
- Hold for a few breaths.
- Inhale and slowly return to face front.
- Switch arms and repeat on the right.

BE MINDFUL

Keep the spine erect. Don't arch your back.

Look over your shoulder.

Maintain slow, steady breathing.

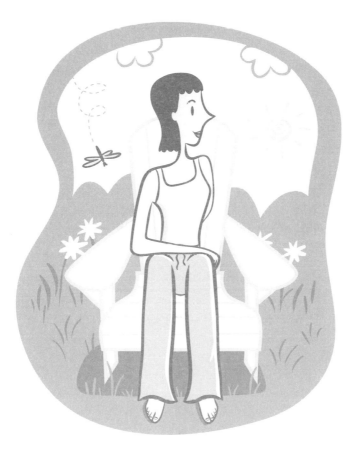

Triangle

Here's waist management for you. The last of the basic postures, the Triangle is a great toner for the waistline and a lateral stretch for your torso and spine. Your arms, back and shoulders get in on the act, too.

- Sit comfortably in Easy Pose.
- Inhale and raise your right arm beside your ear. Your left arm should be on the arm of the chair.
- Exhale and bend to your left. Your body forms a straight line diagonally from your fingertips to your waist. If you really want to get into it, look upward at your right hand.
- Inhale and return to center.
- Switch arms and repeat on other side.

BE MINDFUL

Keep your arm overhead in a straight line.

Keep your buttocks on the chair.

Point your fingertips.

Don't twist or curl your body.

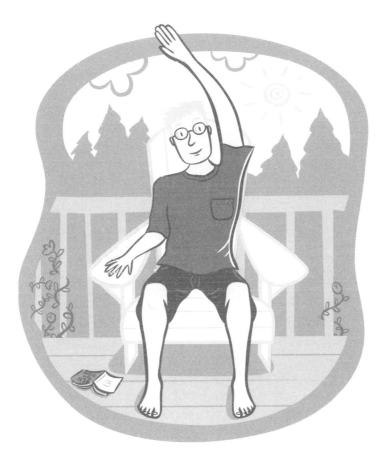

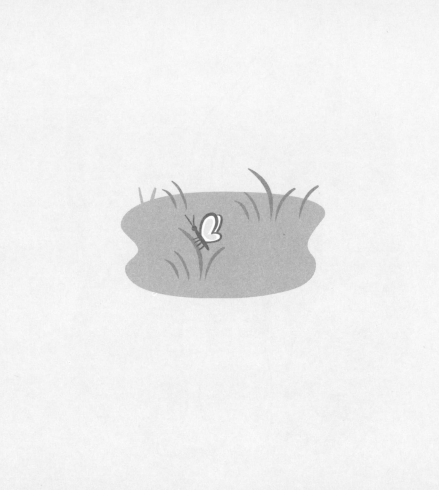

Meditation

Meditation

There's a lot of chatter going on inside our brains. Sometimes it's impossible to shut it up. It keeps us up at night. Causes frown lines and worry lines galore. Enter meditation. For this brief time, forget work. Forget the kids. In fact, forget yourself. Meditation is a time we give ourselves. If you're indoors, put the phone on hold. If outdoors, leave the cellphone indoors.

Meditation may sound like a religious rite or an illusory practice. In fact, it is neither. It is simply the practice of centering one's attention for the purpose of calming the mind through concentration. It's really about being with yourself in silence and stillness. There are many ways to meditate. The most important thing to keep in mind when selecting a style of meditation is to keep it simple. We have three forms of meditation for you. Something for everyone, from simply breathing to listening to music to focusing on an object such as a candle — one of our favorites. Try not to burn down the cottage!

In our over-active lives, there seems to be little time for meditation. To many people, it may sound like a waste of time. However, setting aside 15 or 20 minutes a day to collect your thoughts is well worth the effort. The best way to start a meditation routine is to sit daily for five or 10 minutes. Gradually lengthen the time in five-minute increments. The benefits of regular meditation include better sleep, increased productivity and a better state of mind.

BE MINDFUL

Practice meditation following the poses and breathing exercises.

Find a quiet place without distractions.

Set a regular time to practice on a daily basis.

Focus on your breathing if you become distracted.

Breathing

Focusing on your breathing is the most simple and accessible style of meditation. Simply sit comfortably with your eyes closed and concentrate on your breathing. Try not to allow any thoughts or concerns to distract you. Throw your laptop out the window. If your mind wanders, bring your attention back to your breathing. By focusing on your breath, you can tune into the silence within yourself.

- Sit comfortably in Easy Pose.
- Exhale completely to the count of eight.
- Inhale slowly to the count of four, feeling your abdomen expand and the air move up through your lungs.
- Exhale to the count of eight, feeling your chest move in slightly and noticing your abdomen contract.
- Keep breathing rhythmic.

BE MINDFUL

Try to keep your facial muscles and body relaxed.

Exhale slowly and evenly.

Focus your attention on your breathing.

Sound

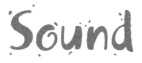

Another form of meditation uses sound or music as the focus of attention. Listening to sound is the easiest form of meditation. The idea of repetitive sound affecting our minds and moods is universal. Drumming, singing, becoming lost in music, has been used to evoke feelings in us for thousands of years — or at least since the sixties. If done regularly, this form of meditation is tremendously relaxing and refreshing.

- Focus your attention on a particular sound, such as a bird singing or soothing music.
- Do not allow your mind to wander from this sound. If your mind wanders, direct it again to the sound, firmly but gently.
- Hold your attention to the sound for three minutes.

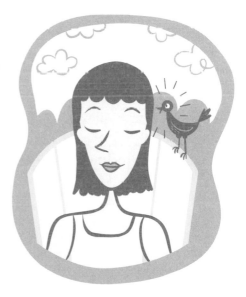

Visual

We can also focus our attention on a visual image or on any pleasing object, such as a flower, a vase or a burning candle flame. In some traditions, people focus on mandalas — geometric patterns that help to calm the mind. The idea is to try to be silent and concentrate on the image and internalize it. By practicing this exercise you will develop concentration, strengthen your eyes and clear your mind.

- Place the object where you can look at it easily.
- Fix your eyes on the object and gaze on it.
- Notice the shape, color and form of the object.
- Try to focus on these aspects of the object and do not allow your mind to wander.
- When your mind wanders from the object, try to return to it gently but firmly.
- Follow this technique at least once a day for three minutes.

CANDLE CONCENTRATION

- Sit comfortably in Easy Pose.

- Place a lit candle about three to four feet away from you on the center of a table, so the flame is about at the level of your chin.

- Gaze at the candle steadily for one minute without blinking.

- Close your eyes, relax your muscles and for one minute visualize the flame in your mind.

- Repeat this sequence up to four times.

- Soon you will be able to hold the image of the flame steady with your eyes closed.

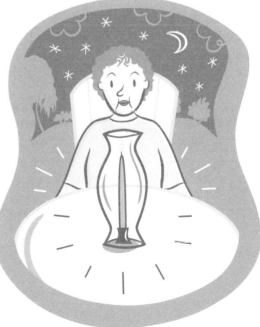

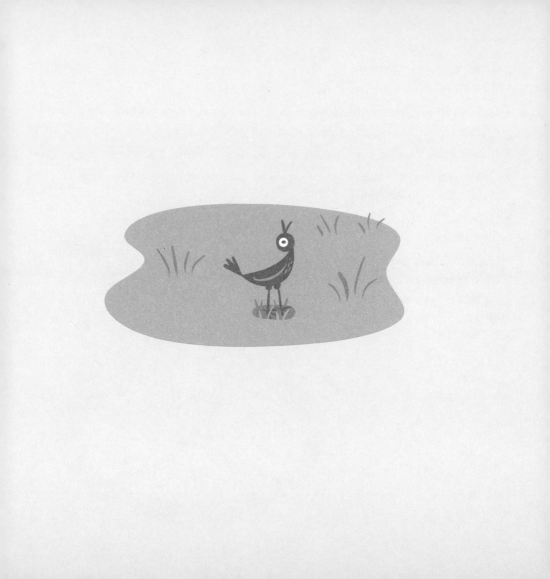

Out of Chair Experience

Out of Chair Experience

There are said to be more than 840,000 yoga postures. And we expect you to learn them all! Once you have mastered the basic positions in the chair, you will be on your way to developing the strength and flexibility needed to do some of these more advanced positions beyond the chair.

The seated positions form a firm foundation for learning other postures. To move forward in your yoga practice, you may want to incorporate several poses that can be done standing or lying down. As you extend your yoga practice to include these new poses, be sure to include a longer relaxation period.

As you become more comfortable in your practice, you may vary your sequence or add new postures. Be sure to continue to spend time with the more familiar poses even as you add new ones.

BE MINDFUL

Remove socks for most postures.

Place a towel or a mat down.

Keep your facial muscles relaxed.

Keep your breathing steady throughout the poses.

If a pose hurts, stop and rest.

After two or three poses, rest for a minute or two.

Cobra

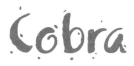

We already introduced you to the Cobra in a chair. This is the original snake charmer. Cobra strengthens the back, abdomen and arms.

- Stretch out on the dock or grass on your stomach. (Put a towel or mat down first if you like.)
- Place your forehead on the ground with the palms of your hands on the ground below your shoulders, your legs and ankles together.
- Inhale and slowly lengthen your neck as you lift your forehead, then slowly arch your back, moving your chest forward and up until you're like a cobra peering out from the top of a snake handler's basket. Expand your chest cavity with each inhalation. Don't lift beyond your belly button.
- Remain in this position for three or four breaths.
- Exhale and slowly lower yourself to the ground, one vertebra at a time, your neck and head unfurling last.

BE MINDFUL

Don't strain. We mean it!

Keep hipbones pressed on the ground.

Relax shoulders and keep them down.

Don't use your arms to push your body up.

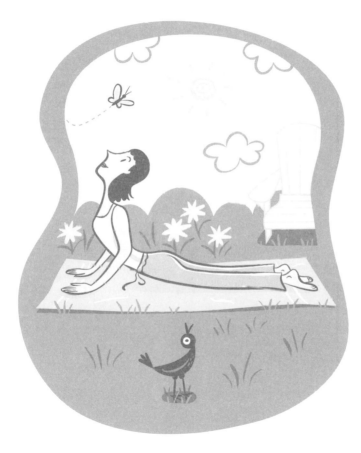

Standing Bend

Massage the internal organs? Yes, we like the sound of that! Digestive and reproductive organs all benefit. The Standing Bend not only establishes a firm foundation for learning other postures, but it helps teach the basic principles of alignment while stretching and strengthening the spine and releasing tension in the lower back. Other benefits include loosening the hamstrings and strengthening the legs.

- Stand with feet together and arms resting alongside your body.
- Inhale and raise your arms above your head, keeping your arms straight and beside your ears.
- Exhale and bend slowly as you stretch your body downwards, bending from your hips and keeping your knees straight.
- Hold your ankles or lower legs, wherever you can grasp comfortably, and bring your forehead as close to your knees as possible.
- Stay in the pose for several breaths.
- Exhale and rise up slowly, vertebra by vertebra, keeping your weight on the balls of your feet.

BE MINDFUL

Make sure your weight is not on your heels.

Keep your knees straight.

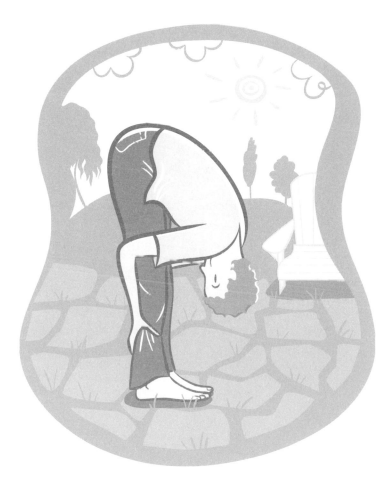

Warrior

The Warrior is a decidedly uncharacteristic name for such a peaceful activity as yoga. But, really, we're all warriors somewhere deep inside. So open your chest and prepare for battle. The Warrior improves balance and strengthens your back, legs, hips, arms and shoulders.

- Stand with feet together and arms resting alongside your body.
- Inhale and raise your arms parallel to the floor, palms facing down.
- Step your right foot to the side about three to four feet. Turn your foot to a 90° angle.
- Your left foot remains grounded and straight.
- Bend your right knee and lower your body into a lunge position over your right foot. Keep your arms at shoulder height, palms facing down.
- Turn your head to the right and look over your right hand.
- Hold the pose for three to six breaths.
- Return to the standing position and repeat on the opposite side.

BE MINDFUL
Be careful if you have knee problems.
Don't allow your bent knee to extend beyond your ankle.

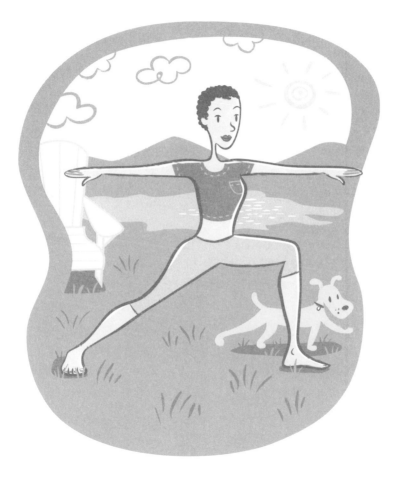

Tree

We love the Tree! As one six-year-old once exclaimed incredulously, "Anyone can do the Tree!" It's a simple but powerful balancing position where, you guessed it, you assume a tree-like pose. At first you may want to stand near the chair or, to be truly sympatico, a tree. This pose improves balance, coordination and circulation.

- Stand with feet together, arms at your side and face relaxed.
- Focus on something stationary in the distance (such as a tree).
- Shift your weight to your left foot.
- Place the sole of your right foot on the inside of your left thigh.
- Place the palms together in front of your chest.
- Hold this position for three to six breaths.
- If you really want to get into it, inhale and move your arms slowly above your head keeping your palms together.
- Exhale and return to starting position.
- Repeat balancing on your right foot.

BE MINDFUL

Don't give up if you start to sway. Even trees sway now and then. Don't press the sole of your foot into your knee.

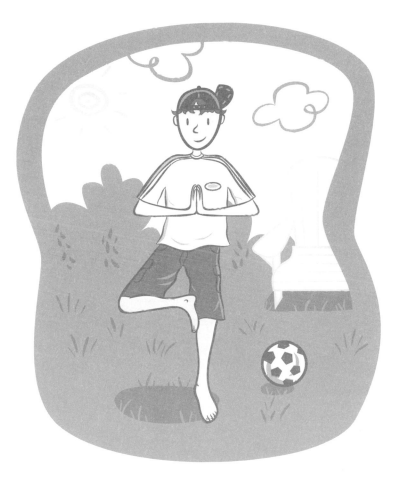

Menus

Here are some sample workout sequences for either energizing or relaxing the body. There's also a quickie that can be done in less than 10 minutes, for those days when you just don't have the time. Whatever the purpose of a particular practice session, it should begin with at least one warm-up and one breathing exercise. Then you can move on to more strenuous poses that strengthen the body and increase endurance.

ENERGIZER
Breath of Fire *p. 18*
Lion Breath *p. 22*
Mountain *p. 28*
Ear Massage *p. 36*
Seated Cobra *p. 50*
Forward Bend *p. 52*
Spinal Twist *p. 54*
Triangle *p. 56*
Seated Relaxation
p. 44

RELAXER
Alternating Breath
p. 16
Cooling Breath *p. 20*
Eye Exercises *p. 34*
Cow *p. 46*
Fish *p. 48*
Forward Bend *p. 52*
Seated Relaxation
p. 44

QUICKIE
Lion Breath *p. 22*
Mountain *p. 28*
Cow *p. 46*
Forward Bend *p. 52*
Seated Relaxation
p. 44

Recommended Reading

Desktop Yoga
by Julie Lusk
Berkeley Publishing
Group 1998

*Pocket Guide to
Hatha Yoga*
by Michele Picozzi
The Crossing Press
1998

Smart Guide to Yoga
by Stephanie
Levin-Gervasi
Cader Books 1999

*Stretching at Your
Computer or Desk*
by Bob Anderson
Shelter Publications
1997

Teach Yourself Yoga
by Mary Stewart
NTC/Contemporary
Publishing Co. 1998

The Little Yoga Book
by Erika Dillman
Warner Books 1999

*The Modern Book of
Yoga: Exercising Mind,
Body and Spirit*
by Anne Kent Rush
Dell Publishing
1996

Yoga & You
by Esther Myers
Random House of
Canada 1996

Yoga Asanas
by Sri Swami
Sivananda
The Divine Life
Society 1993

Yoga for Beginners
by Harry Waesse
Sterling Publishing
Co. 1995

Yoga Mind & Body
by Sivananda Yoga
Vedenta Center
Dorling Kindersley
1998

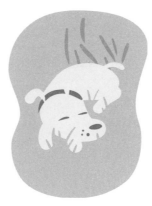